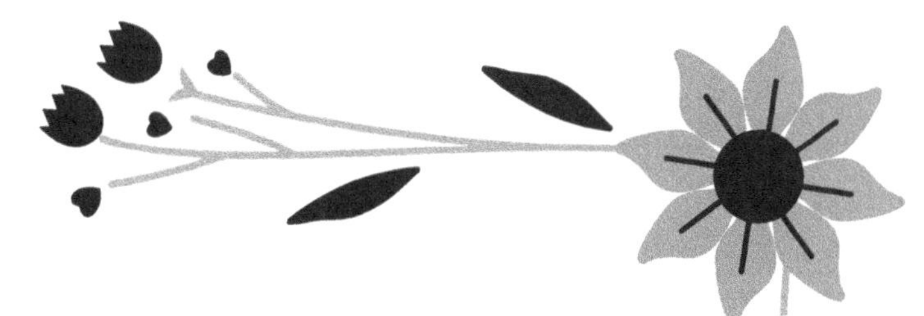

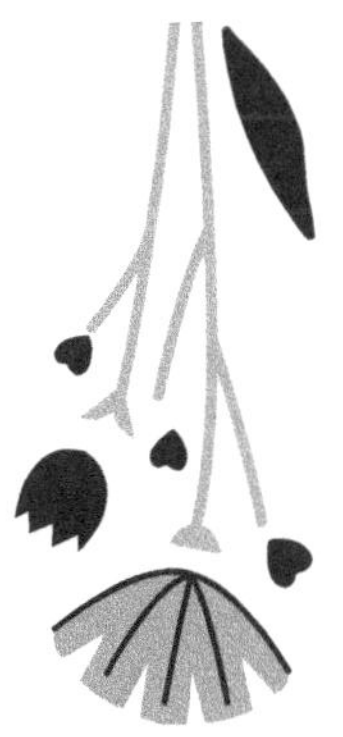

This belongs to:

____

I Dedicate this Empowerment Journal To YOU.

You are Fearfully and Wonderfully Made! Never let people define who you are. You determine that. Whatever you do, do not ever compare yourself to others. Focus on becoming the best version of yourself. Be sure to spend some time with you because YOU matter too!

I wish you much success and love on your
self-love journey.
-Ulaonda Parham, M.A.Ed.

Self-Love Affirmations

I AM NOT MY PAST

I AM FREE

I AM NOT MY TRAUMA

I AM THANKFUL

MEMORY LANE

"Jesus Christ is the same Yesterday and today and forever." Hebrew 13.8 NIV

1. As you walk down memory lane, ask yourself, do you want to go? Was your response lets go, I don't want to go, or was it a little of both? Write down your thoughts below...

____

____

____

____

____

____

____

2. After answering question number one, how do you feel?

____

____

____

____

____

____

____

3. Write down ALL your emotions, define each one.

4. Did you understand the definitions of your feelings? Were you surprised?

5. Before answering the questions above, did you avoid going down your memory lane? Why or Why not?

____

____

____

____

____

____

____

6. Study the scripture reference Hebrew 13:8. What are the words saying to you when you read this?

____

____

____

____

____

____

7. How can you intentionally apply Hebrew 13:8 to your life? (take your time, this is your journey)

8. Was Hebrew 13:8 comforting, convicting, or neither? Explain...

Self-Love Affirmations

MY MENTAL WELLNESS IS A PRIORITY
I CAN EAT HEALTHIER/EXERCISE
I CAN REST MORE
I SHOULD LAUGH MORE

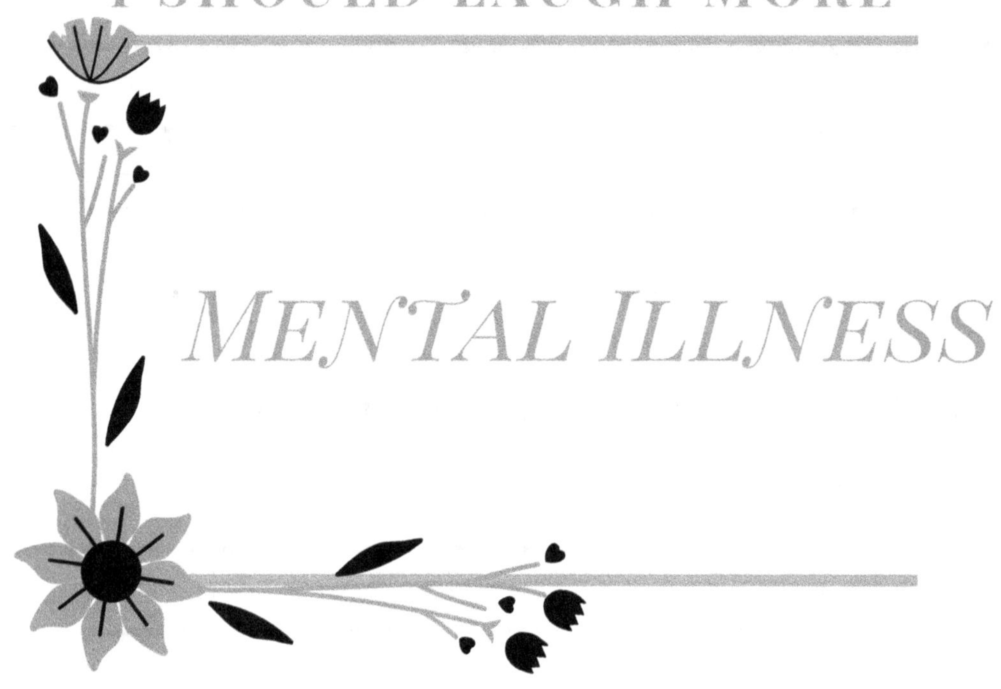

"I have told you these things so that in me you may have peace in this world you will have trouble. But take heart I have overcome the World."
John 16:33 NIV

1. Define mental illness.

2. What does mental illness mean to you?

3. Do you feel comfortable with taking a mental health questionnaire?

(Disclaimer: this is not a medical accurate test;
it is only used for self-awareness)
If you answered Yes, the website is listed below:
https://screening.mhanational.org/screening-tools

If you answered No, that is okay! Take it whenever you are ready)

If you answered Yes, what do the results mean to you? Discuss...

____

____

____

____

____

____

____

____

____

____

____

____

4. According to your results, do you feel that you Need TO SEEK HELP? If your answer was yes, are you ok with seeing a therapist/counselor? Why or Why not?

____

____

____

____

____

____

____

____

5. How are counselors and therapists different/similar?

____

____

____

____

____

____

____

6. How comfortable are you with speaking about mental illnesses? Circle: comfortable somewhat comfortable not comfortable. Why?

____

____

____

____

____

____

____

7. How comfortable are you with speaking about mental illnesses? Circle: comfortable somewhat comfortable not comfortable. Why?

____

____

____

____

____

____

____

**8. Study the scripture reference John 16:33 What
are the words saying to you when you read this?**

____

____

____

____

____

____

____

**9. How can you intentionally apply John 16:33 to your
life?**

____

____

____

____

____

____

____

10. Was John 16:33 comforting, convicting, or neither? Explain...

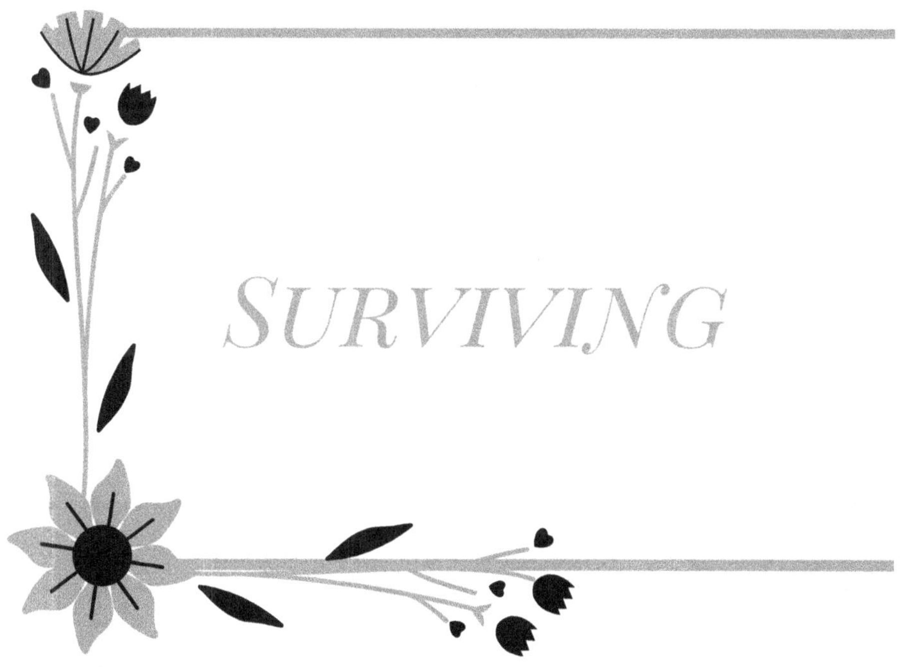

*"This is what the Lord says: the people
Who survive the sword will find favor in
the wilderness; I will come to give rest to Israel."*
Jeremiah 31:2 NIV

1. Define survival.

____

____

____

____

____

____

____

____

2. Describe your survival journey?

____

____

____

____

____

____

____

**3. Was it difficult for you to reflect on survival?
Why or why not?**

____

____

____

____

____

____

____

4. What does it mean to cope?

____

____

____

____

____

____

____

5. Define the four major coping mechanisms. Give examples of each.

Problem-focused-

____

____

____

____

____

____

Emotion-focused-

____

____

____

____

____

____

Meaning-focused-

____

____

____

____

____

____

____

____

Social coping- (support seeking)

____

____

____

____

____

____

____

____

6. List some of your coping mechanisms. (Be honest this is your unique journey, and you should be proud of your resilience)

____

____

____

____

____

____

____

7. Did you experience childhood trauma? if so, have you triumphed over your trauma: or have you intentionally avoided your trauma experiences? (it is your journey...answer whenever you are ready to have this conversation with yourself.)

____

____

____

____

____

____

____

8. Study the scripture reference Jeremiah 31:2. What are the words saying to you when you read this?

____

____

____

____

____

____

____

9. How can you intentionally apply Jeremiah 31:2 to your life?

____

____

____

____

____

____

____

10. Was Jeremiah 31:2 comforting, convicting, or neither? Explain...

Self-Love Affirmations

I forgive me

My body/mind can be healed

I am powerful

I will shift my mindset

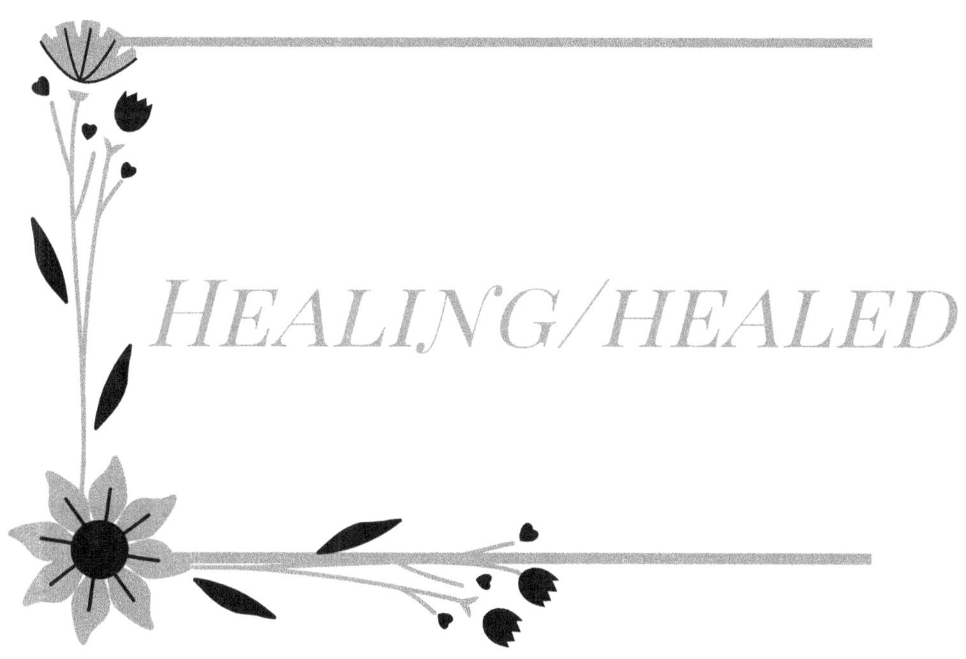

Healing/healed

*"Behold I will bring it health and cure, and
I will cure them, and will reveal unto them the
abundance of peace and truth."*
Jeremiah 33:6 KJV

1. Have you or anyone close to you been physically or mentally ill? Describe your experiences.

____

____

____

____

____

____

____

2. Do you believe faith alone can heal you? Why or why not?

____

____

____

____

____

____

**3. Is it possible to be healed by a combination of
God, medicine, and a healthy diet? Explain...**

____

____

____

____

____

____

____

**4. Study the scripture reference Jeremiah 33:6. What
are the words saying to you when you read this?**

____

____

____

____

____

____

____

5. How can you intentionally apply Jeremiah 33:6 to your life?

____

____

____

____

____

____

6. Was Jeremiah 33:6 comforting, convicting, or neither? Explain...

____

____

____

____

____

____

SELF-LOVE AFFIRMATIONS

I AM SUCCESSFUL

FAITH OVER FEARS

TRUST THE PROCESS

I AM WORTH IT

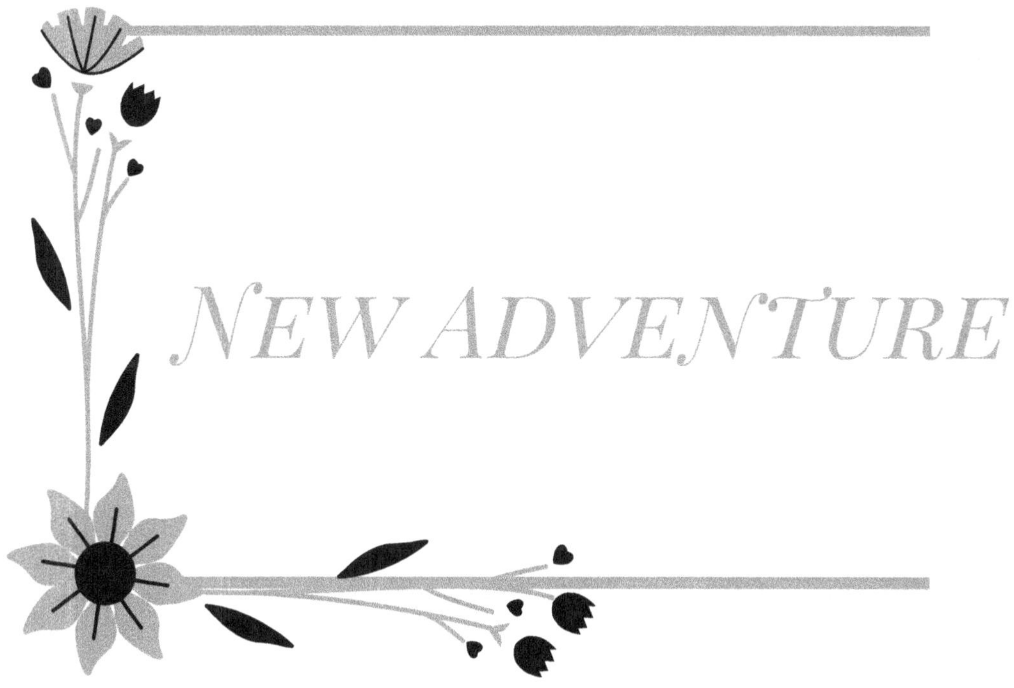

"Have not I commanded thee? Be strong
and of good courage. Be not afraid,
neither be though dismayed: For the Lord
Thy God is with thee whithersoever thou goest."
Joshua 1:9 KJV

1. Are you in your comfort zone? Are you happy there? Explain...

____

____

____

____

____

____

____

2. Make a list of your goals...

____

____

____

____

____

____

____

3. Have you achieved any of your goals? Did you achieve any in your comfort zone? How? If not are you okay with this? Explain...

4. Make a list of your fears. (be honest with you)

**5. Your list of fears represents what "stepping out"
of your comfort zone looks like. Do you agree or
disagree? Explain...**

____

____

____

____

____

____

____

**6. Study the scripture reference Joshua 1:9. What are
the words saying to you when you read this?**

____

____

____

____

____

____

____

7. How can you intentionally apply Joshua 1:9 to your life?

____

____

____

____

____

____

____

8. Was Joshua 1:9 comforting, convicting, or neither? Explain...

____

____

____

____

____

____

____

SELF-LOVE AFFIRMATIONS

MY FEELINGS ARE VALID

I GIVE MYSELF TIME TO GRIEVE

MY PAIN IS TEMPORARY

I HAVE MORE REASONS TO SMILE

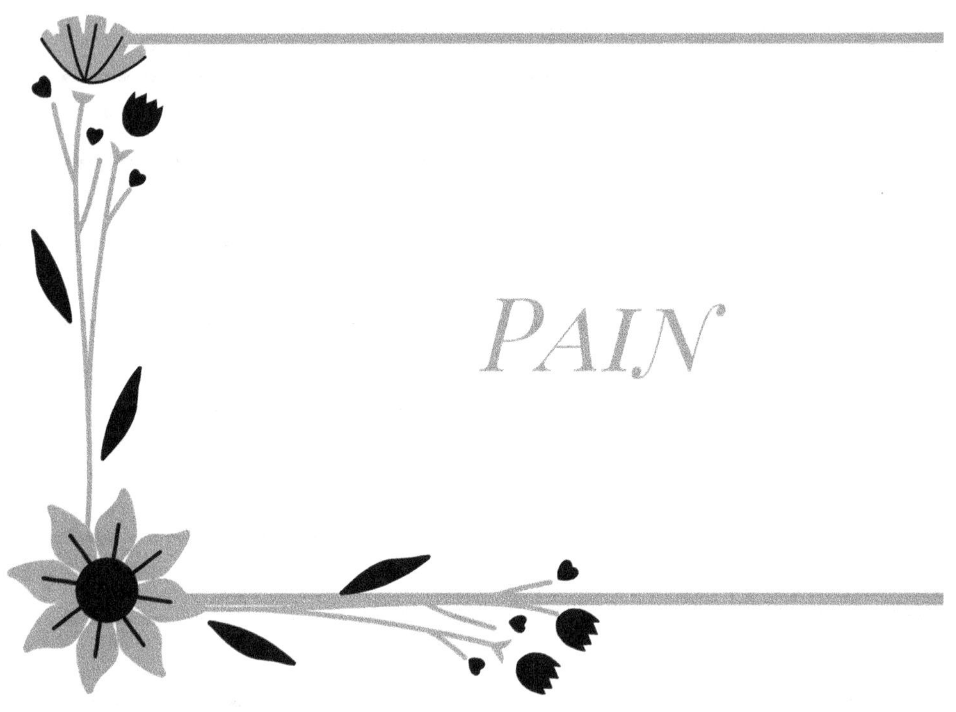

PAIN

"And God shall wipe away all tears from their eyes; and there shall be no more death, neither sorrow, nor crying, neither shall there be any more pain: for the former things are passed away." Revelation 21:4 KJV

1. Have you experienced pain or are you experiencing pain? Write down your painful experiences.

____

____

____

____

____

____

____

____

2. Was it difficult? Did you skip number one?

(If so, it is okay. Give yourself time. Identifying pain is an important part of your healing journey.)

If you wrote down your painful moments, make a list of your feelings. Do you understand your feelings? Share your thoughts

____

____

____

____

____

____

____

3. Are you okay? _____ Pain is a tough topic to talk about... Give yourself time. Take a break... Remember acknowledging pain or any feelings is progress. This is your unique journey. Do what you need to do to cope.
If your answer was yes, share your experiences on reaching such a difficult breakthrough.

____

____

____

____

____

____

____

4. List some ways that you cope when dealing with pain? Be true to yourself!

____

____

____

____

____

____

5. Have you ever experienced grief from the death of a loved one? Did you get grief support?

____

____

____

____

____

____

____

____

6. Did you turn to alcohol, drugs, sex, food, work, exercise, prayer, journaling, meditation, counseling, friends/family, or etc? Circle all that apply. How do you feel about your choice(s) of coping mechanisms? Did they help? Explain...

____

____

____

____

____

____

____

7. Did you turn to God? Did you get closer to God? Do you believe in God? Did you find God? Are you mad at God? Did you turn away from God? Discuss your answers.

____

____

____

____

____

____

____

8. Study the scripture reference Revelation 21:4. What are the words saying to you when you read this?

____

____

____

____

____

____

____

9. How can you intentionally apply Revelation 21:4 to your life?

____

____

____

____

____

____

____

10. Was Revelation 21:4 comforting, convicting, or neither? Explain...

____

____

____

____

____

____

____

Self-Love Affirmations

I LOVE ME

I AM IMPERFECT…AND THAT'S OK

I AM ENOUGH

I CHOOSE LOVE OVER HATE

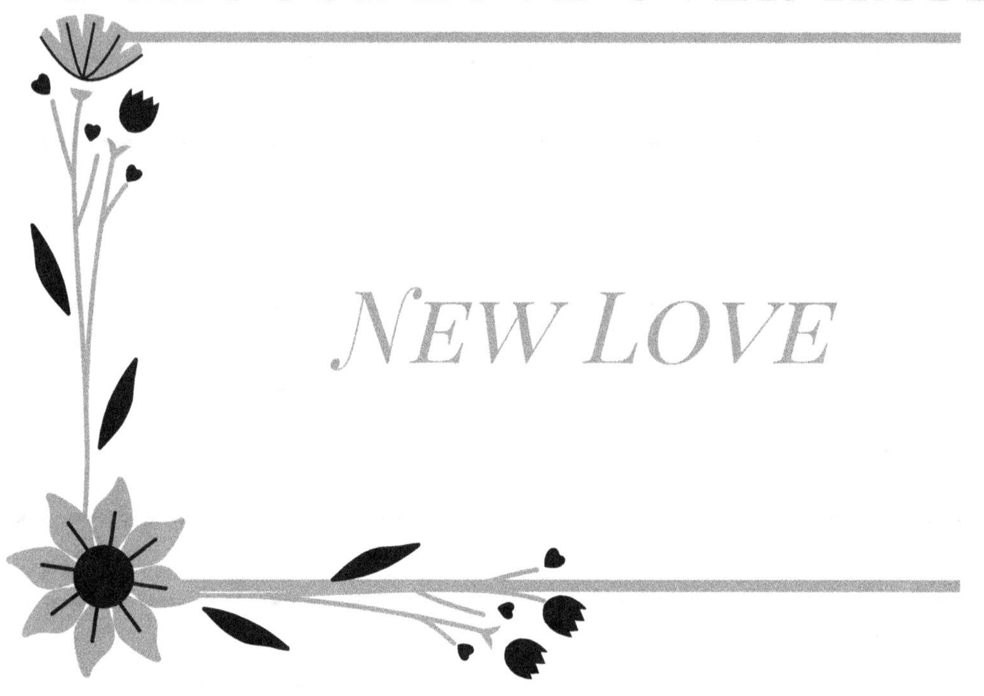

New Love

"Above all,
love each other deeply, because love covers
over a multitude of sins." 1 Peter 4:8 NIV

1. Define love.

2. Make a list of some things you love. **Do them!

3. What are some of the "surprise" experiences you had in your life? What are some things you told yourself that you would never do, but you did it?

____

____

____

____

____

____

____

4. What are some of the "unwanted" surprises that happened to you in your life? Have you grown from them?

____

____

____

____

____

____

____

5. If you are a single parent or was raised by a single parent; do you feel broken or that you failed? Describe your thoughts. (remember all your feelings are valid and important) Express yourself...

____

____

____

____

____

____

____

6. Are you influenced by social media/society's expectations for your life? Are you okay with your answer? Explain...

____

____

____

____

____

____

____

7. Have you ever felt as if you were living in someone else's shadow? As if you did not know who you were because you were living to family and friends' expectations. How does this make you feel? List some ways that you can switch the focus to yourself instead?

____

____

____

____

____

____

____

____

8. What are some ways that you can focus on individualizing your beliefs? How can you embrace your ideas and implement them in your life?

____

____

____

____

____

____

____

9. Study the scripture reference 1 Peter 4:8. What are the words saying to you when you read this?

---

10. How can you intentionally apply 1 Peter 4:8 to your life?

Self-Love Affirmations

I AM A FIGHTER

I AM A CHILD OF A KING

I AM CONTENT

I WILL NEVER GIVE UP

Strength

"I can do all things through Christ which strengthenth me." Philippians 4:13 KJV

1. Define strength.

____

____

____

____

____

____

____

____

2. Do you consider yourself strong? Why or why not?

____

____

____

____

____

____

____

3. Is there a connection between your pain and strength? Explain...

____

____

____

____

____

____

____

4. Do you think strength is a good characteristic to have? Explain...

____

____

____

____

____

____

____

5. Write down some ways you consider yourself strong.

6. If your list was short, do you think this makes you weak? Why or why not?

7. Make a list of your strengths/weaknesses.

____

____

____

____

____

____

____

**8. Rate yourself based on your thoughts on where you
stand regarding strength in each of these areas. Discuss
your answers...**
Mentally 1 2 3 4 5 6 7 8 9 10
Spiritually 1 2 3 4 5 6 7 8 9 10
Physically 1 2 3 4 5 6 7 8 9 10
Financially 1 2 3 4 5 6 7 8 9 10

____

____

____

____

____

____

9. Write down strategies you will work on to improve your ratings

____

____

____

____

____

____

____

____

10. Study the scripture reference Philippians 4:13. What are the words saying to you when you read this?

____

____

____

____

____

____

____

11. How can you intentionally apply Philippians 4:13 to your life?

____

____

____

____

____

____

____

12. Was Philippians 4:13 comforting, convicting, or neither? Explain...

____

____

____

____

____

____

____

SELF-LOVE AFFIRMATIONS

I BELIEVE IN ME

I AM CAPABLE

I LIVE BY FAITH...NOT BY SIGHT

I TRUST GOD

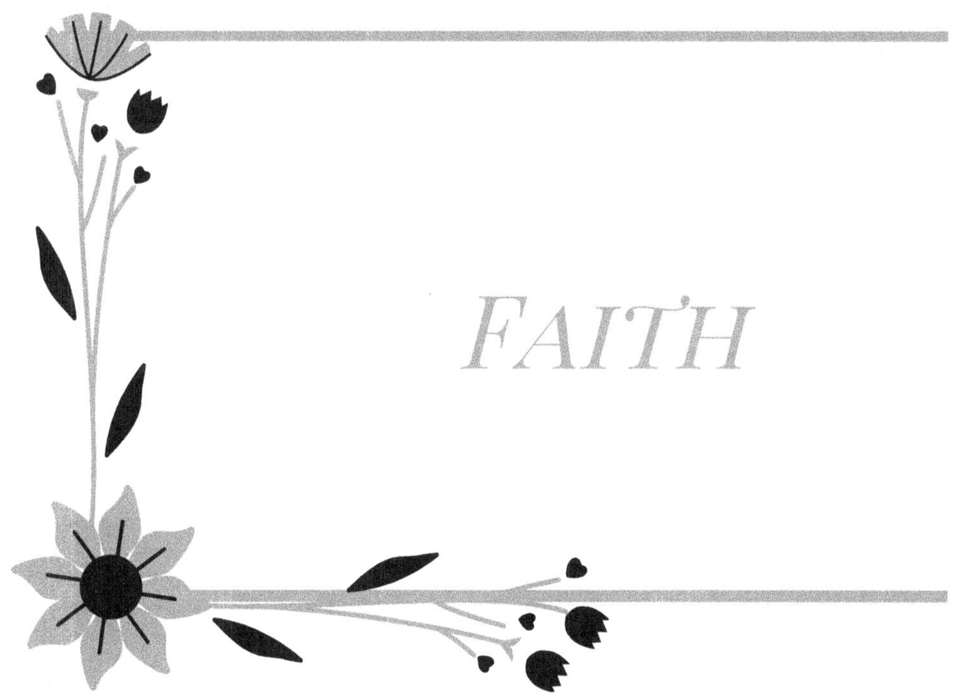

FAITH

"For we walk by faith, not by sight."
2 Corinthians 5:7 KJV

1. Define faith.

____

____

____

____

____

____

____

2. What is your definition of faith?

____

____

____

____

____

____

____

3. Do you think you can have faith and not be spiritual or believe in God? Explain...

____

____

____

____

____

____

4. Do you think it is good to have faith in people? Why or Why not?

____

____

____

____

____

____

5. How can you increase your faith?

____

____

____

____

____

____

____

____

**6. Is there a connection between patience and faith?
Explain...**

____

____

____

____

____

____

____

7. List some ways that you can improve your patience.

____

____

____

____

____

____

____

8. What does the term "testing your faith" mean to you?

____

____

____

____

____

____

____

9. Study the scripture reference 2 Corinthians 5:7. What are the words saying to you when you read this?

____

____

____

____

____

____

____

10. How can you intentionally apply 2 Corinthians 5:7 to life?

____

____

____

____

____

____

11. Was 2 Corinthians 5:7 comforting, convicting, or neither? Explain...

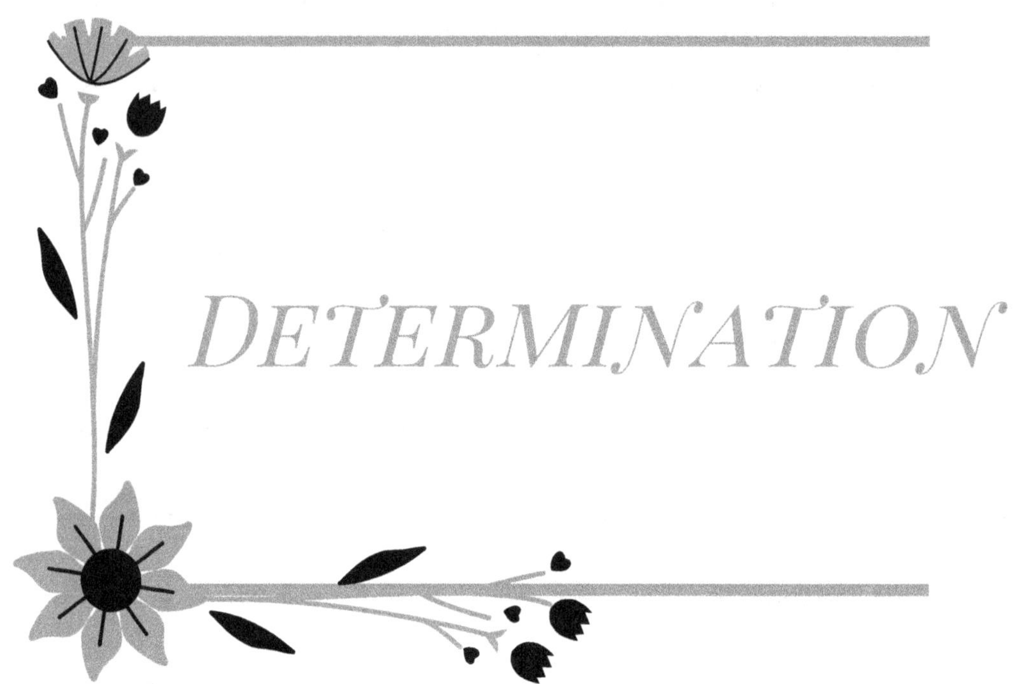

SELF-LOVE AFFIRMATIONS

I AM MY BIGGEST CHEERLEADER

I DESERVE TO REACH MY GOALS

I WANT THE BEST FOR ME

I GOT THIS

DETERMINATION

"For I know the thoughts that I think towards you. saith the Lord, thoughts of peace, and not of evil, to give you an expected end."
Jeremiah 29:11 KJV

1. Define determination.

2. What does it mean to have self-determination? Do you consider yourself to be a determined person? Are you okay with your answer? Explain...

3. What are goals and why are they important?

____

____

____

____

____

____

____

____

**4. Make a list of all the goals you have had in your
lifetime. Place a check on all of the ones you have
achieved, underline the ones you are working on, and
circle the ones that are no longer your goals.**

____

____

____

____

____

____

____

5. What are some of the factors that have kept you from reaching your goals?

____

____

____

____

____

____

____

6. Do you lack confidence, knowledge, or motivation to reach your goals? If your answer was yes, do you believe there is a solution to your answer?

____

____

____

____

____

____

____

7. Do you feel that you are worthy of achieving your goals? Explain..

---

8. Define motivation? Do you see a connection with determination? Explain...

---

9. Study the scripture reference Jeremiah 29:11. What are the words saying to you when you read this?

____

____

____

____

____

____

____

10. How can you intentionally apply Jeremiah 29:11 to life?

____

____

____

____

____

____

____

11. Was Jeremiah 29:11 comforting, convicting, or neither? Explain...

SELF-LOVE AFFIRMATIONS

I HOLD MYSELF ACCOUNTABLE

I WILL PREPARE FOR MY/FAMILY FUTURE

I WILL ADJUST TO CHANGE

PREPARATION

"The Lord is my shepherd...
Psalm 23 1-6 KJV

1. Define preparation.

____

____

____

____

____

____

____

2. What does it mean "to prepare"? How important is it to you to prepare for the unexpected? (ex. Repairs, death, sickness) Explain...

____

____

____

____

____

____

____

**3. What are some ways you prepare for you and
your family?**

____

____

____

____

____

____

____

4. Are all preparations good? Why or why not?

____

____

____

____

____

____

____

5. Make a list of preparations you would like to prepare for...

____

____

____

____

____

____

____

____

6. Do you have life insurance? Why or why not?

____

____

____

____

____

____

____

7. How can you be intentional about preparing for your death? Write out a plan of action.

____

____

____

____

____

____

____

8. Study the scripture reference Psalm 23 1-6. What are the words saying to you when you read this?

____

____

____

____

____

____

____

9. How can you intentionally apply Psalm 23 1-6 to life?

____

____

____

____

____

____

____

10. Was Psalm 23 1-6 comforting, convicting, or neither? Explain...

____

____

____

____

____

____

____

SELF-LOVE AFFIRMATIONS

I AM CALM/RELAXED

EXERCISE IS GOOD FOR MY MIND

I WILL LET GO OF THE THINGS I CANNOT CONTROL

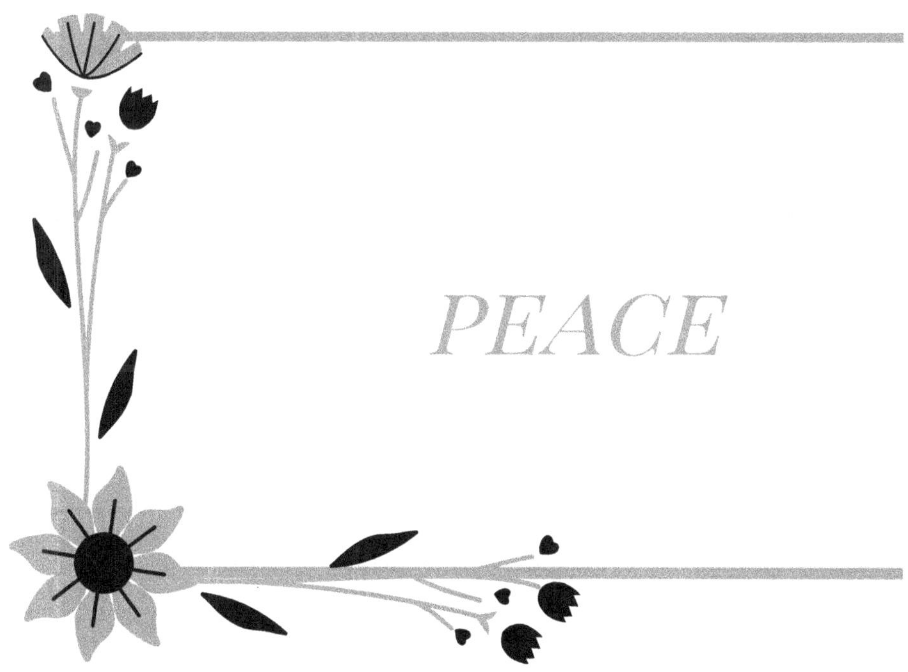

"Peace I leave with you, my peace I give unto you: not as the world giveth, give I unto you. Let not your heart be troubled, neither let it be afraid."
John 14:27 KJV

1. Define peace.

2. Are you currently at peace? Describe this feeling...

3. What are some ways you obtain peace?

____

____

____

____

____

____

____

4. How do you maintain your peaceful state of mind?

____

____

____

____

____

____

5. Make a list of things that brought/bring you peace?

____

____

____

____

____

____

____

6. What are some things that interfere with your peace? (try to avoid if possible)

____

____

____

____

____

____

____

7. What does "guard your heart" mean? What are some ways that you can be more intentional about guarding your heart?

____

____

____

____

____

____

____

8. Make a list of the things that you CAN control in your life.

____

____

____

____

____

____

____

9. Make a list of the things you CANNOT control in your life.

Note: Be intentional with not allowing those things
that you cannot control to interfere with
disturbing your peace. (I personally pray in advance for God
to help prepare me mentally, physically, emotionally,
and financially for these uncontrollable things.)

____

____

____

____

____

____

____

____

10. Study the scripture reference John 14:27. What are the words saying to you when you read this?

____

____

____

____

____

____

11. How can you intentionally apply Psalm 23 1-6 to life?

____

____

____

____

____

____

____

12. Was Psalm 23 1-6 comforting, convicting, or neither? Explain...

____

____

____

____

____

____

____

Journal Prompts

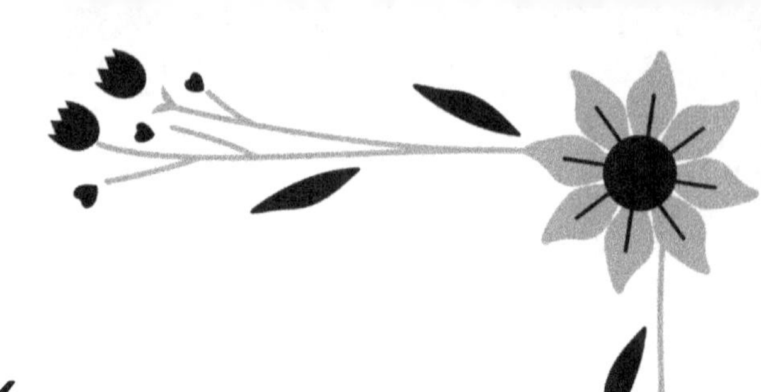

1. If I could talk to my younger self, what would I say?
2. Make a list of at least 20 things that make me smile.
3. Who am I? Describe yourself using at least 15 words.
4. Make a list of at least 20 things that make me angry.
5. I'm so sick of...
6. What activities make me calm...
7. When I'm in pain (emotional, physical, mental), what is the nicest thing I can do for myself...
8. I am thankful for...
9. What is a habit that I love most?
10. What keeps me awake at night?
11. Write a thank you letter to someone...
12. My dream career looks like?
13. How do I deal with anger?
14. Am I comfortable with being alone?
15. What will make the world a better place?

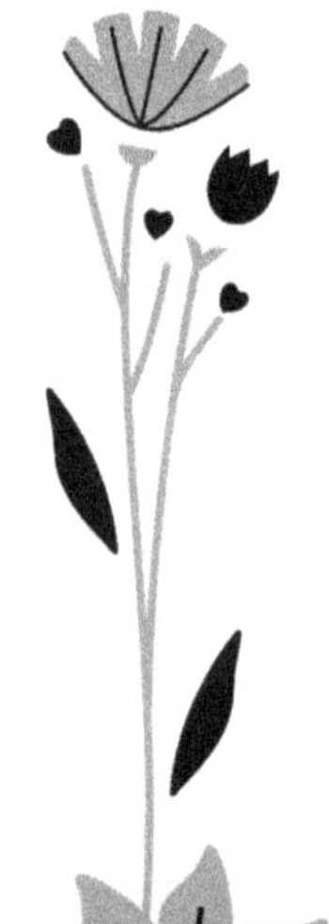

Journal Prompts

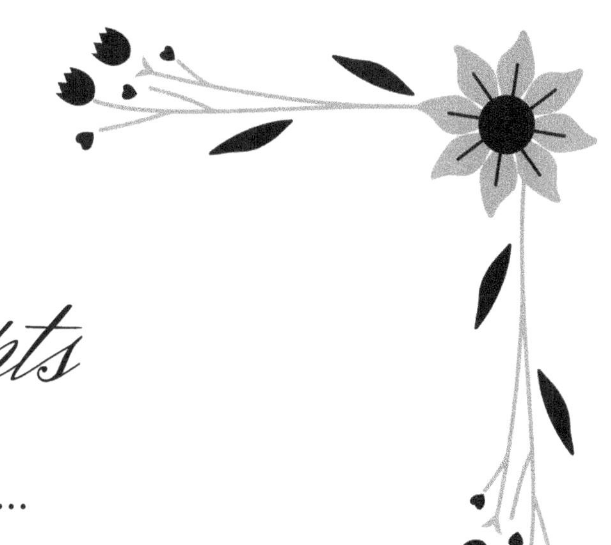

16. I am most confident when...

17. What is unique about me?

18. I need more...

19. What parts of my life need improving?

20. What is bothering me right now?

21. I can love myself more by...

22. If I were given $100,000, I would...

23. What self-love habit do I want to start?

24. How does being abandoned affect me?

25. What brings me joy?

26. How do I handle conflict?

27. If I could open up a business, what would it be?

28. Write me a thank you letter...

29. How do I recharge?

30. What am I interested in learning more about?

31. Write about my favorite animal...

32. What helps me slow down?

33. How can I be more present for myself/family?

34. How do I put myself first without feeling guilty?

35. How do I advocate for myself?

Journal Prompts

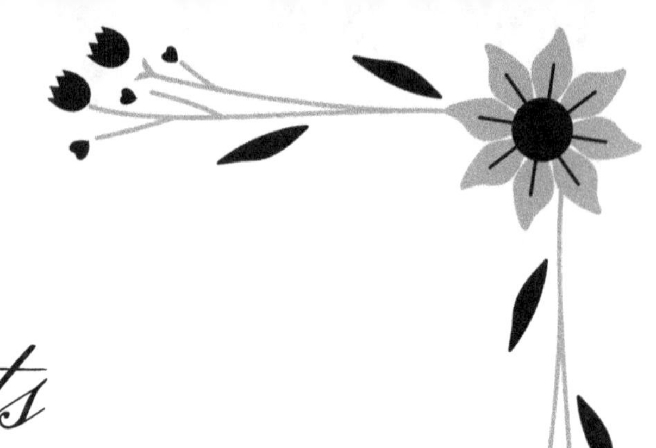

36. Make a list of 10 things that make me cry...

37. My most important boundaries are...

38. How do I protect my boundaries?

39. How do I stay focused and steer clear of distractions?

40. Write about a teacher or coach who has inspired me...

41. What is the best part of quarantine?

42. What is the worst part of quarantine?

43. What do I need to do more of?

44. Do I have a childhood trauma that I never healed f from?

45. Name one thing that I look forward to each day?

46. What is a habit that I dislike the most?

47. What habit do I need to incorporate into my life?

48. What does my anxiety feel like?

49. I will never forget this moment in my life...

50. How do I embrace my authentic self, even when it looks different?

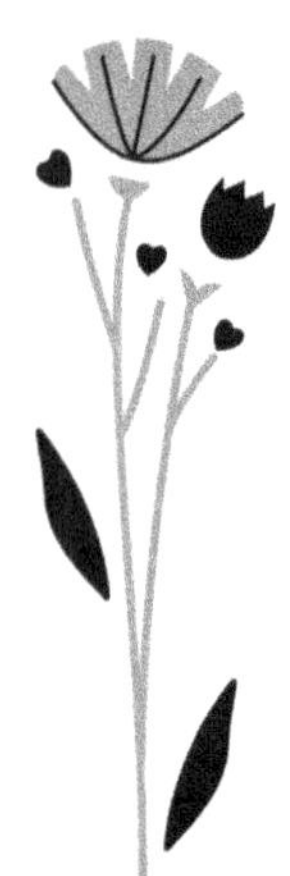

Date:

Date:

Date:

Date:

Date:

Date:

Date:

Date:

Date:

Date:

Date: